Date: _____   Weight: _____

Starting measurements:

Measurements	
Neck	
Chest	
Bicep	
Waist	
Hips	
Thigh	
Calf	

Other stats to track :

_____

_____

_____

_____

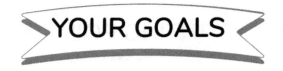

YOUR GOALS

Weight: _____

Your dream measurements:

Measurements	
Neck	
Chest	
Bicep	
Waist	
Hips	
Thigh	
Calf	

Other stats :

_____
_____
_____

☆ ☆ ☆ ☆ ☆

FITNESS TRACKER

Meals

Time	Items	Serving	Cals	Sugar	Protein	Fiber	Carbs	Fat
Totals								

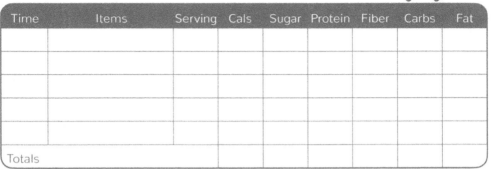

Exercise

Exercise	Set 1	Set 2	Set 3	Set 4	Set 5	Set 6

Water Tracker

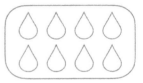

Notes:

Measurements

Measurements	
Neck	
Chest	
Bicep	
Waist	
Hips	
Thigh	
Calf	

Cardio

Exercise	Time	Intensity	Cals

FITNESS TRACKER

Meals

Time	Items	Serving	Cals	Sugar	Protein	Fiber	Carbs	Fat
Totals								

Exercise

Water Tracker

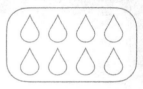

Exercise	Set 1	Set 2	Set 3	Set 4	Set 5	Set 6

Notes:

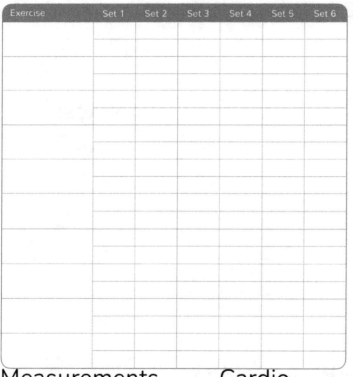

Measurements

Cardio

Measurements	
Neck	
Chest	
Bicep	
Waist	
Hips	
Thigh	
Calf	

Exercise	Time	Intensity	Cals

FITNESS TRACKER

Meals

Time	Items	Serving	Cals	Sugar	Protein	Fiber	Carbs	Fat
Totals								

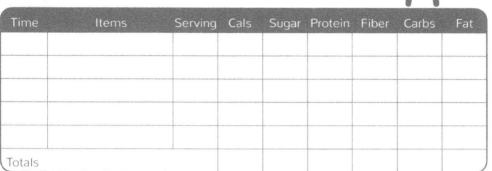

Exercise

Exercise	Set 1	Set 2	Set 3	Set 4	Set 5	Set 6

Water Tracker

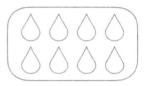

Notes:

Measurements

Measurements	
Neck	
Chest	
Bicep	
Waist	
Hips	
Thigh	
Calf	

Cardio

Exercise	Time	Intensity	Cals

FITNESS TRACKER

Meals

Time	Items	Serving	Cals	Sugar	Protein	Fiber	Carbs	Fat
Totals								

Exercise

Exercise	Set 1	Set 2	Set 3	Set 4	Set 5	Set 6

Water Tracker

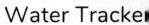

Notes:

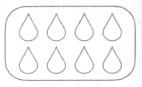

Measurements

Measurements	
Neck	
Chest	
Bicep	
Waist	
Hips	
Thigh	
Calf	

Cardio

Exercise	Time	Intensity	Cals

FITNESS TRACKER

Meals

Time	Items	Serving	Cals	Sugar	Protein	Fiber	Carbs	Fat
Totals								

Exercise

Exercise	Set 1	Set 2	Set 3	Set 4	Set 5	Set 6

Water Tracker

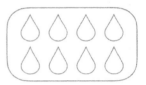

Notes:

Measurements

Measurements	
Neck	
Chest	
Bicep	
Waist	
Hips	
Thigh	
Calf	

Cardio

Exercise	Time	Intensity	Cals

FITNESS TRACKER
Meals

Time	Items	Serving	Cals	Sugar	Protein	Fiber	Carbs	Fat
Totals								

Exercise

Water Tracker

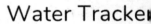

Exercise	Set 1	Set 2	Set 3	Set 4	Set 5	Set 6

Notes:

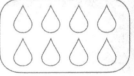

Measurements

Cardio

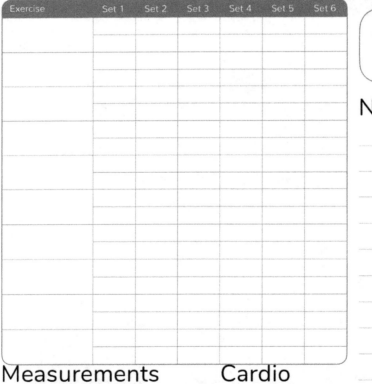

Measurements	
Neck	
Chest	
Bicep	
Waist	
Hips	
Thigh	
Calf	

Exercise	Time	Intensity	Cals

FITNESS TRACKER
Meals

Time	Items	Serving	Cals	Sugar	Protein	Fiber	Carbs	Fat
Totals								

Exercise

Water Tracker

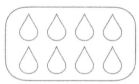

Exercise	Set 1	Set 2	Set 3	Set 4	Set 5	Set 6

Notes:

Measurements

Cardio

Measurements	
Neck	
Chest	
Bicep	
Waist	
Hips	
Thigh	
Calf	

Exercise	Time	Intensity	Cals

WEEKLY NOTES

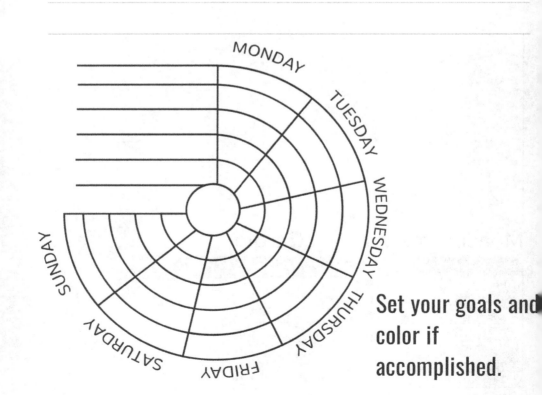

Set your goals and color if accomplished.

FITNESS TRACKER
Meals

Time	Items	Serving	Cals	Sugar	Protein	Fiber	Carbs	Fat
Totals								

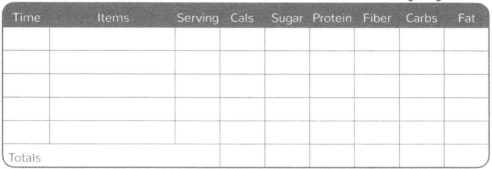

Exercise

Exercise	Set 1	Set 2	Set 3	Set 4	Set 5	Set 6

Water Tracker

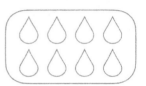

Notes:

Measurements

Measurements	
Neck	
Chest	
Bicep	
Waist	
Hips	
Thigh	
Calf	

Cardio

Exercise	Time	Intensity	Cals

FITNESS TRACKER

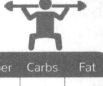

Meals

Time	Items	Serving	Cals	Sugar	Protein	Fiber	Carbs	Fat
Totals								

Exercise

Exercise	Set 1	Set 2	Set 3	Set 4	Set 5	Set 6

Water Tracker

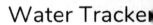

Notes:

_____
_____
_____
_____
_____
_____
_____
_____
_____
_____
_____
_____
_____

Measurements

Measurements	
Neck	
Chest	
Bicep	
Waist	
Hips	
Thigh	
Calf	

Cardio

Exercise	Time	Intensity	Cals

FITNESS TRACKER
Meals

Time	Items	Serving	Cals	Sugar	Protein	Fiber	Carbs	Fat
Totals								

Exercise

Water Tracker

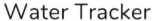

Exercise	Set 1	Set 2	Set 3	Set 4	Set 5	Set 6

Notes:

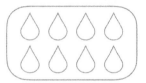

Measurements

Cardio

Measurements	
Neck	
Chest	
Bicep	
Waist	
Hips	
Thigh	
Calf	

Exercise	Time	Intensity	Cals

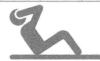

FITNESS TRACKER
Meals

Time	Items	Serving	Cals	Sugar	Protein	Fiber	Carbs	Fat
Totals								

Exercise

Water Tracker

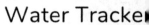

Exercise	Set 1	Set 2	Set 3	Set 4	Set 5	Set 6

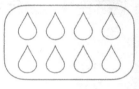

Notes:

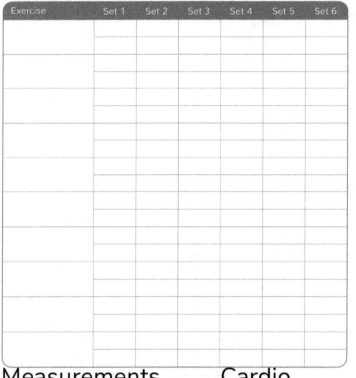

Measurements   Cardio

Measurements	
Neck	
Chest	
Bicep	
Waist	
Hips	
Thigh	
Calf	

Exercise	Time	Intensity	Cals

FITNESS TRACKER
Meals

Time	Items	Serving	Cals	Sugar	Protein	Fiber	Carbs	Fat
Totals								

Exercise

Water Tracker

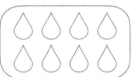

Exercise	Set 1	Set 2	Set 3	Set 4	Set 5	Set 6

Notes:

Measurements   Cardio

Measurements	
Neck	
Chest	
Bicep	
Waist	
Hips	
Thigh	
Calf	

Exercise	Time	Intensity	Cals

FITNESS TRACKER

Meals

Time	Items	Serving	Cals	Sugar	Protein	Fiber	Carbs	Fat
Totals								

Exercise

Exercise	Set 1	Set 2	Set 3	Set 4	Set 5	Set 6

Water Tracker

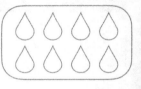

Notes:

Measurements

Measurements	
Neck	
Chest	
Bicep	
Waist	
Hips	
Thigh	
Calf	

Cardio

Exercise	Time	Intensity	Cals

FITNESS TRACKER
Meals

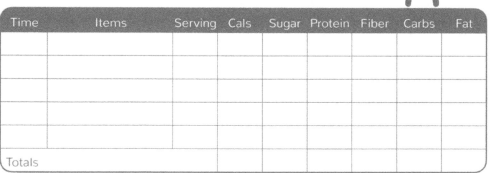

Time	Items	Serving	Cals	Sugar	Protein	Fiber	Carbs	Fat
Totals								

Exercise

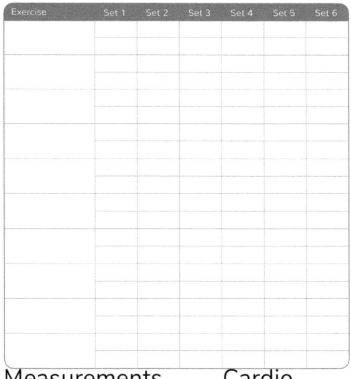

Exercise	Set 1	Set 2	Set 3	Set 4	Set 5	Set 6

Water Tracker

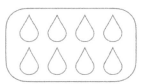

Notes:

Measurements

Measurements	
Neck	
Chest	
Bicep	
Waist	
Hips	
Thigh	
Calf	

Cardio

Exercise	Time	Intensity	Cals

WEEKLY NOTES

Set your goals and color if accomplished.

FITNESS TRACKER

Meals

Time	Items	Serving	Cals	Sugar	Protein	Fiber	Carbs	Fat
Totals								

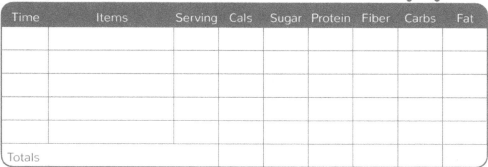

Exercise

Exercise	Set 1	Set 2	Set 3	Set 4	Set 5	Set 6

Water Tracker

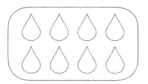

Notes:

Measurements

Measurements	
Neck	
Chest	
Bicep	
Waist	
Hips	
Thigh	
Calf	

Cardio

Exercise	Time	Intensity	Cals

FITNESS TRACKER
Meals

Time	Items	Serving	Cals	Sugar	Protein	Fiber	Carbs	Fat
Totals								

Exercise

Water Tracker

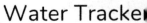

Exercise	Set 1	Set 2	Set 3	Set 4	Set 5	Set 6

Notes:

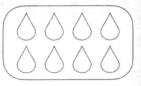

Measurements

Measurements	
Neck	
Chest	
Bicep	
Waist	
Hips	
Thigh	
Calf	

Cardio

Exercise	Time	Intensity	Cals

FITNESS TRACKER
Meals

Time	Items	Serving	Cals	Sugar	Protein	Fiber	Carbs	Fat
Totals								

Exercise

Exercise	Set 1	Set 2	Set 3	Set 4	Set 5	Set 6

Water Tracker

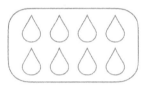

Notes:

Measurements

Measurements	
Neck	
Chest	
Bicep	
Waist	
Hips	
Thigh	
Calf	

Cardio

Exercise	Time	Intensity	Cals

FITNESS TRACKER

Meals

Time	Items	Serving	Cals	Sugar	Protein	Fiber	Carbs	Fat
Totals								

Exercise

Exercise	Set 1	Set 2	Set 3	Set 4	Set 5	Set 6

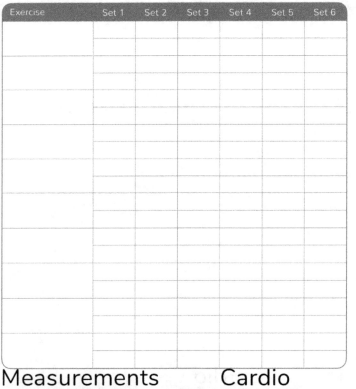

Water Tracker

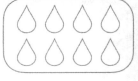

Notes:

Measurements

Measurements	
Neck	
Chest	
Bicep	
Waist	
Hips	
Thigh	
Calf	

Cardio

Exercise	Time	Intensity	Cals

FITNESS TRACKER
Meals

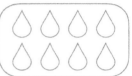

Time	Items	Serving	Cals	Sugar	Protein	Fiber	Carbs	Fat
Totals								

Exercise

Water Tracker

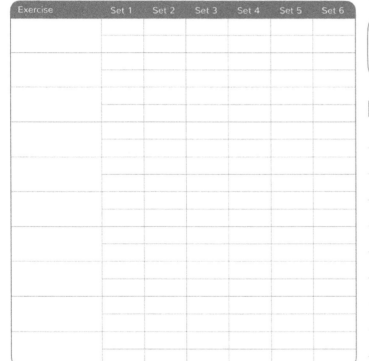

Exercise	Set 1	Set 2	Set 3	Set 4	Set 5	Set 6

Notes:

Measurements

Measurements	
Neck	
Chest	
Bicep	
Waist	
Hips	
Thigh	
Calf	

Cardio

Exercise	Time	Intensity	Cals

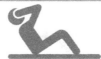

FITNESS TRACKER

Meals

Time	Items	Serving	Cals	Sugar	Protein	Fiber	Carbs	Fat
Totals								

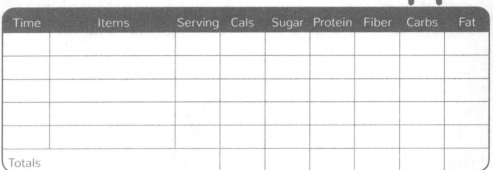

Exercise

Exercise	Set 1	Set 2	Set 3	Set 4	Set 5	Set 6

Water Tracker

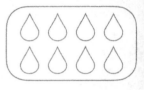

Notes:

Measurements

Measurements	
Neck	
Chest	
Bicep	
Waist	
Hips	
Thigh	
Calf	

Cardio

Exercise	Time	Intensity	Cals

FITNESS TRACKER

Meals

Time	Items	Serving	Cals	Sugar	Protein	Fiber	Carbs	Fat
Totals								

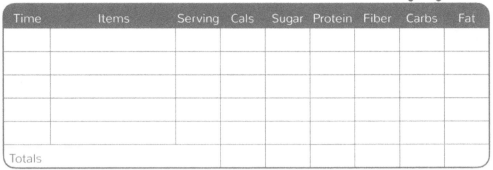

Exercise

Exercise	Set 1	Set 2	Set 3	Set 4	Set 5	Set 6

Water Tracker

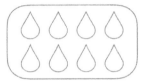

Notes:

Measurements

Measurements	
Neck	
Chest	
Bicep	
Waist	
Hips	
Thigh	
Calf	

Cardio

Exercise	Time	Intensity	Cals

WEEKLY NOTES

Set your goals and color if accomplished.

FITNESS TRACKER

Meals

Time	Items	Serving	Cals	Sugar	Protein	Fiber	Carbs	Fat
Totals								

Exercise

Water Tracker

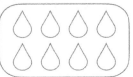

Exercise	Set 1	Set 2	Set 3	Set 4	Set 5	Set 6

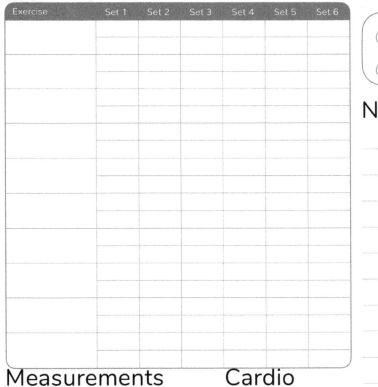

Notes:

Measurements

Measurements	
Neck	
Chest	
Bicep	
Waist	
Hips	
Thigh	
Calf	

Cardio

Exercise	Time	Intensity	Cals

FITNESS TRACKER
Meals

Time	Items	Serving	Cals	Sugar	Protein	Fiber	Carbs	Fat
Totals								

Exercise

Exercise	Set 1	Set 2	Set 3	Set 4	Set 5	Set 6

Water Tracker

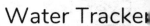

Notes:

Measurements

Measurements	
Neck	
Chest	
Bicep	
Waist	
Hips	
Thigh	
Calf	

Cardio

Exercise	Time	Intensity	Cals

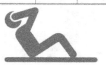

FITNESS TRACKER

Meals

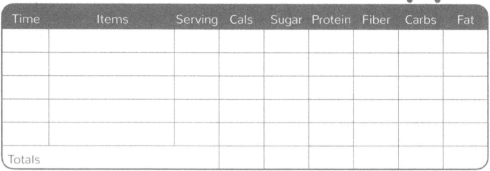

Time	Items	Serving	Cals	Sugar	Protein	Fiber	Carbs	Fat
Totals								

Exercise

Exercise	Set 1	Set 2	Set 3	Set 4	Set 5	Set 6

Water Tracker

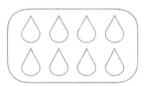

Notes:

Measurements

Measurements	
Neck	
Chest	
Bicep	
Waist	
Hips	
Thigh	
Calf	

Cardio

Exercise	Time	Intensity	Cals

FITNESS TRACKER

Meals

Time	Items	Serving	Cals	Sugar	Protein	Fiber	Carbs	Fat
Totals								

Exercise

Water Tracker

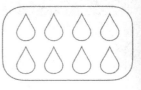

Notes:

Exercise	Set 1	Set 2	Set 3	Set 4	Set 5	Set 6

Measurements

Cardio

Measurements	
Neck	
Chest	
Bicep	
Waist	
Hips	
Thigh	
Calf	

Exercise	Time	Intensity	Cals

FITNESS TRACKER

Meals

Time	Items	Serving	Cals	Sugar	Protein	Fiber	Carbs	Fat
Totals								

Exercise

Exercise	Set 1	Set 2	Set 3	Set 4	Set 5	Set 6

Water Tracker

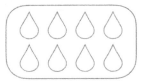

Notes:

Measurements

Measurements	
Neck	
Chest	
Bicep	
Waist	
Hips	
Thigh	
Calf	

Cardio

Exercise	Time	Intensity	Cals

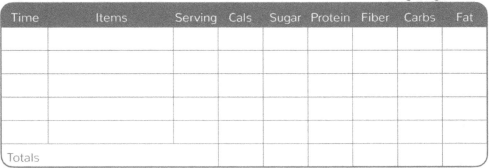
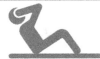

FITNESS TRACKER
Meals

Time	Items	Serving	Cals	Sugar	Protein	Fiber	Carbs	Fat
Totals								

Exercise

Water Tracker

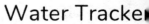

Exercise	Set 1	Set 2	Set 3	Set 4	Set 5	Set 6

Notes:

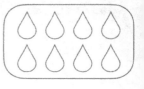

Measurements

Cardio

Measurements	
Neck	
Chest	
Bicep	
Waist	
Hips	
Thigh	
Calf	

Exercise	Time	Intensity	Cals

FITNESS TRACKER
Meals

Time	Items	Serving	Cals	Sugar	Protein	Fiber	Carbs	Fat
Totals								

Exercise

Exercise	Set 1	Set 2	Set 3	Set 4	Set 5	Set 6

Water Tracker

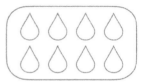

Notes:

Measurements

Measurements	
Neck	
Chest	
Bicep	
Waist	
Hips	
Thigh	
Calf	

Cardio

Exercise	Time	Intensity	Cals

WEEKLY NOTES

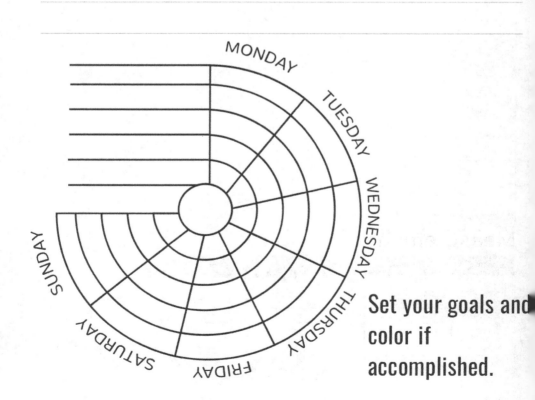

Set your goals and color if accomplished.

FITNESS TRACKER
Meals

Time	Items	Serving	Cals	Sugar	Protein	Fiber	Carbs	Fat
Totals								

Exercise

Exercise	Set 1	Set 2	Set 3	Set 4	Set 5	Set 6

Water Tracker

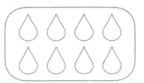

Notes:

Measurements

Measurements	
Neck	
Chest	
Bicep	
Waist	
Hips	
Thigh	
Calf	

Cardio

Exercise	Time	Intensity	Cals

FITNESS TRACKER
Meals

Time	Items	Serving	Cals	Sugar	Protein	Fiber	Carbs	Fat
Totals								

Exercise

Water Tracker

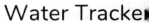

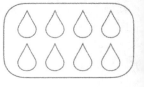

Notes:

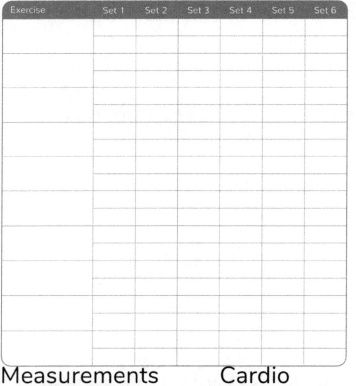

Measurements

Cardio

Measurements	
Neck	
Chest	
Bicep	
Waist	
Hips	
Thigh	
Calf	

Exercise	Time	Intensity	Cals

FITNESS TRACKER
Meals

Time	Items	Serving	Cals	Sugar	Protein	Fiber	Carbs	Fat
Totals								

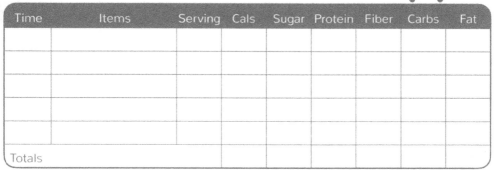

Exercise

Exercise	Set 1	Set 2	Set 3	Set 4	Set 5	Set 6

Water Tracker

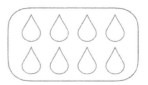

Notes:

Measurements

Measurements	
Neck	
Chest	
Bicep	
Waist	
Hips	
Thigh	
Calf	

Cardio

Exercise	Time	Intensity	Cals

FITNESS TRACKER
Meals

Time	Items	Serving	Cals	Sugar	Protein	Fiber	Carbs	Fat
Totals								

Exercise

Water Tracker

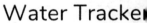

Exercise	Set 1	Set 2	Set 3	Set 4	Set 5	Set 6

Notes:

Measurements

Cardio

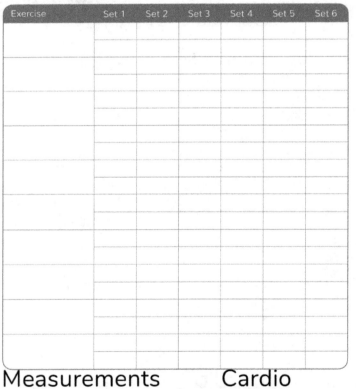

Measurements	
Neck	
Chest	
Bicep	
Waist	
Hips	
Thigh	
Calf	

Exercise	Time	Intensity	Cals

FITNESS TRACKER

Meals

Time	Items	Serving	Cals	Sugar	Protein	Fiber	Carbs	Fat
Totals								

Exercise

Exercise	Set 1	Set 2	Set 3	Set 4	Set 5	Set 6

Water Tracker

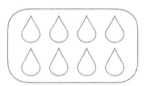

Notes:

Measurements

Measurements	
Neck	
Chest	
Bicep	
Waist	
Hips	
Thigh	
Calf	

Cardio

Exercise	Time	Intensity	Cals

FITNESS TRACKER

Meals

Time	Items	Serving	Cals	Sugar	Protein	Fiber	Carbs	Fat
Totals								

Exercise

Exercise	Set 1	Set 2	Set 3	Set 4	Set 5	Set 6

Water Tracker

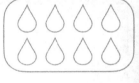

Notes:

Measurements

Measurements	
Neck	
Chest	
Bicep	
Waist	
Hips	
Thigh	
Calf	

Cardio

Exercise	Time	Intensity	Cals

FITNESS TRACKER
Meals

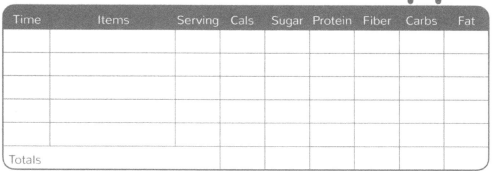

Time	Items	Serving	Cals	Sugar	Protein	Fiber	Carbs	Fat
Totals								

Exercise

Water Tracker

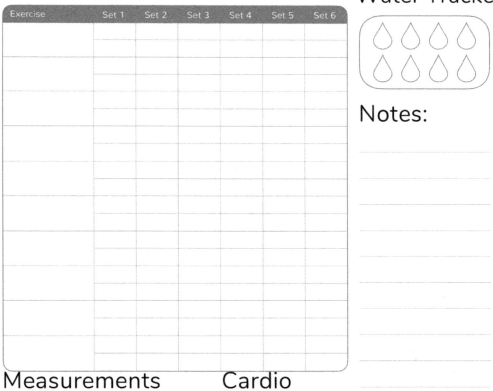

Exercise	Set 1	Set 2	Set 3	Set 4	Set 5	Set 6

Notes:

Measurements

Measurements	
Neck	
Chest	
Bicep	
Waist	
Hips	
Thigh	
Calf	

Cardio

Exercise	Time	Intensity	Cals

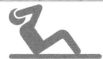

WEEKLY NOTES

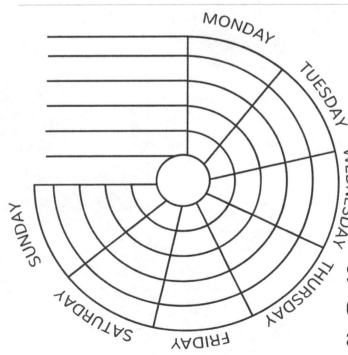

Set your goals and color if accomplished.

FITNESS TRACKER
Meals

Time	Items	Serving	Cals	Sugar	Protein	Fiber	Carbs	Fat
Totals								

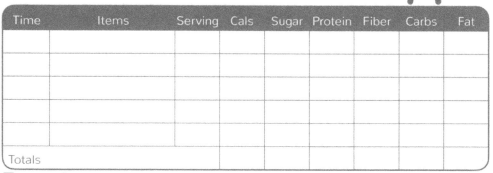

Exercise

Exercise	Set 1	Set 2	Set 3	Set 4	Set 5	Set 6

Water Tracker

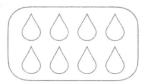

Notes:

Measurements

Measurements	
Neck	
Chest	
Bicep	
Waist	
Hips	
Thigh	
Calf	

Cardio

Exercise	Time	Intensity	Cals

FITNESS TRACKER

Meals

Time	Items	Serving	Cals	Sugar	Protein	Fiber	Carbs	Fat
Totals								

Exercise

Water Tracker

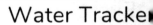

Exercise	Set 1	Set 2	Set 3	Set 4	Set 5	Set 6

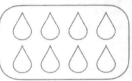

Notes:

Measurements

Cardio

Measurements	
Neck	
Chest	
Bicep	
Waist	
Hips	
Thigh	
Calf	

Exercise	Time	Intensity	Cals

FITNESS TRACKER

Meals

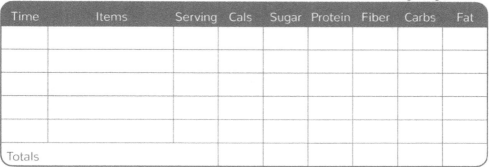

Time	Items	Serving	Cals	Sugar	Protein	Fiber	Carbs	Fat
Totals								

Exercise

Exercise	Set 1	Set 2	Set 3	Set 4	Set 5	Set 6

Water Tracker

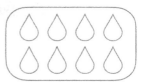

Notes:

Measurements

Measurements	
Neck	
Chest	
Bicep	
Waist	
Hips	
Thigh	
Calf	

Cardio

Exercise	Time	Intensity	Cals

FITNESS TRACKER

Meals

Time	Items	Serving	Cals	Sugar	Protein	Fiber	Carbs	Fat
Totals								

Exercise

Exercise	Set 1	Set 2	Set 3	Set 4	Set 5	Set 6

Water Tracker

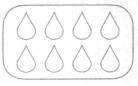

Notes:

Measurements

Measurements	
Neck	
Chest	
Bicep	
Waist	
Hips	
Thigh	
Calf	

Cardio

Exercise	Time	Intensity	Cals

FITNESS TRACKER

Meals

Time	Items	Serving	Cals	Sugar	Protein	Fiber	Carbs	Fat
Totals								

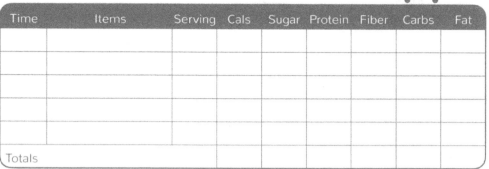

Exercise

Exercise	Set 1	Set 2	Set 3	Set 4	Set 5	Set 6

Water Tracker

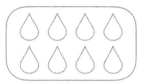

Notes:

Measurements

Measurements	
Neck	
Chest	
Bicep	
Waist	
Hips	
Thigh	
Calf	

Cardio

Exercise	Time	Intensity	Cals

FITNESS TRACKER

Meals

Time	Items	Serving	Cals	Sugar	Protein	Fiber	Carbs	Fat
Totals								

Exercise

Water Tracker

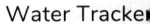

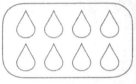

Notes:

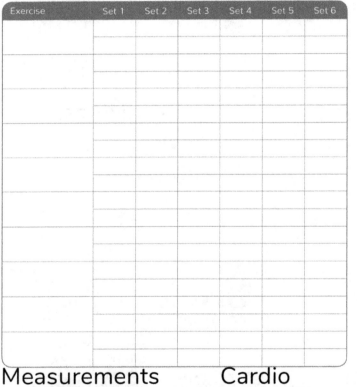

Exercise	Set 1	Set 2	Set 3	Set 4	Set 5	Set 6

Measurements

Cardio

Measurements	
Neck	
Chest	
Bicep	
Waist	
Hips	
Thigh	
Calf	

Exercise	Time	Intensity	Cals

FITNESS TRACKER

Meals

Time	Items	Serving	Cals	Sugar	Protein	Fiber	Carbs	Fat
Totals								

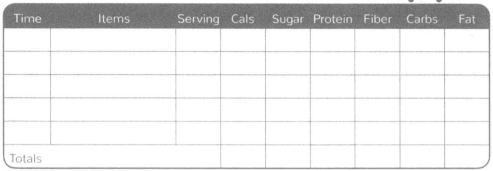

Exercise

Exercise	Set 1	Set 2	Set 3	Set 4	Set 5	Set 6

Water Tracker

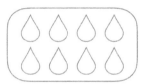

Notes:

Measurements

Measurements	
Neck	
Chest	
Bicep	
Waist	
Hips	
Thigh	
Calf	

Cardio

Exercise	Time	Intensity	Cals

WEEKLY NOTES

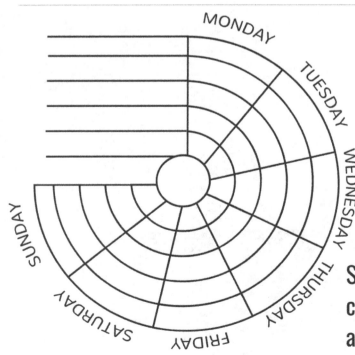

Set your goals and color if accomplished.

FITNESS TRACKER
Meals

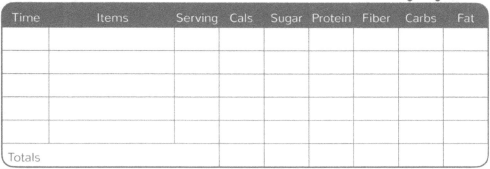

Time	Items	Serving	Cals	Sugar	Protein	Fiber	Carbs	Fat
Totals								

Exercise

Exercise	Set 1	Set 2	Set 3	Set 4	Set 5	Set 6

Water Tracker

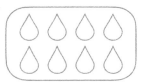

Notes:

_____
_____
_____
_____
_____
_____
_____
_____
_____
_____
_____
_____

Measurements

Measurements	
Neck	
Chest	
Bicep	
Waist	
Hips	
Thigh	
Calf	

Cardio

Exercise	Time	Intensity	Cals

FITNESS TRACKER

Meals

Time	Items	Serving	Cals	Sugar	Protein	Fiber	Carbs	Fat
Totals								

Exercise

Exercise	Set 1	Set 2	Set 3	Set 4	Set 5	Set 6

Water Tracker

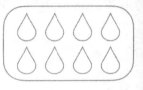

Notes:

Measurements

Measurements	
Neck	
Chest	
Bicep	
Waist	
Hips	
Thigh	
Calf	

Cardio

Exercise	Time	Intensity	Cals

FITNESS TRACKER
Meals

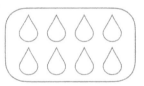

Time	Items	Serving	Cals	Sugar	Protein	Fiber	Carbs	Fat
Totals								

Exercise

Water Tracker

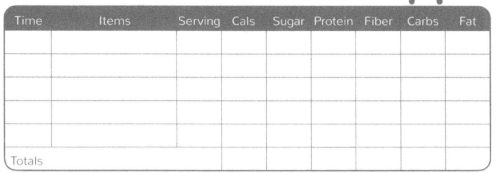

Exercise	Set 1	Set 2	Set 3	Set 4	Set 5	Set 6

Notes:

Measurements

Cardio

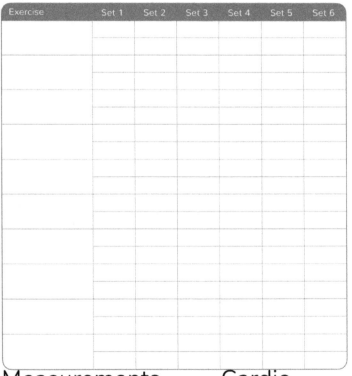

Measurements	
Neck	
Chest	
Bicep	
Waist	
Hips	
Thigh	
Calf	

Exercise	Time	Intensity	Cals

FITNESS TRACKER

Meals

Time	Items	Serving	Cals	Sugar	Protein	Fiber	Carbs	Fat
Totals								

Exercise

Exercise	Set 1	Set 2	Set 3	Set 4	Set 5	Set 6

Water Tracker

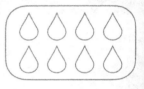

Notes:

Measurements

Measurements	
Neck	
Chest	
Bicep	
Waist	
Hips	
Thigh	
Calf	

Cardio

Exercise	Time	Intensity	Cals

FITNESS TRACKER
Meals

Time	Items	Serving	Cals	Sugar	Protein	Fiber	Carbs	Fat
Totals								

Exercise

Exercise	Set 1	Set 2	Set 3	Set 4	Set 5	Set 6

Water Tracker

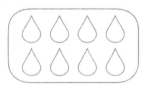

Notes:

Measurements

Measurements	
Neck	
Chest	
Bicep	
Waist	
Hips	
Thigh	
Calf	

Cardio

Exercise	Time	Intensity	Cals

FITNESS TRACKER

Meals

Time	Items	Serving	Cals	Sugar	Protein	Fiber	Carbs	Fat
Totals								

Exercise

Water Tracker

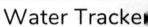

Exercise	Set 1	Set 2	Set 3	Set 4	Set 5	Set 6

Notes:

Measurements

Measurements	
Neck	
Chest	
Bicep	
Waist	
Hips	
Thigh	
Calf	

Cardio

Exercise	Time	Intensity	Cals

FITNESS TRACKER

Meals

Time	Items	Serving	Cals	Sugar	Protein	Fiber	Carbs	Fat
Totals								

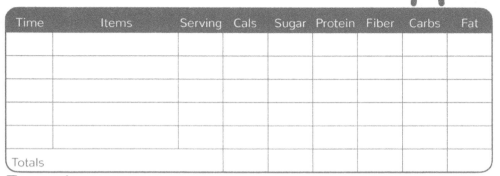

Exercise

Exercise	Set 1	Set 2	Set 3	Set 4	Set 5	Set 6

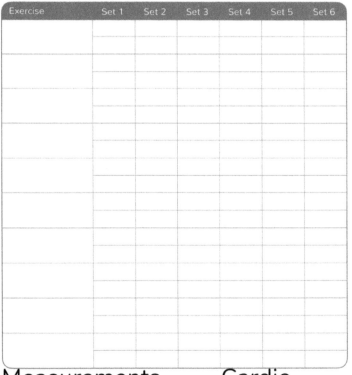

Water Tracker

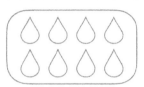

Notes:

Measurements

Measurements	
Neck	
Chest	
Bicep	
Waist	
Hips	
Thigh	
Calf	

Cardio

Exercise	Time	Intensity	Cals

WEEKLY NOTES

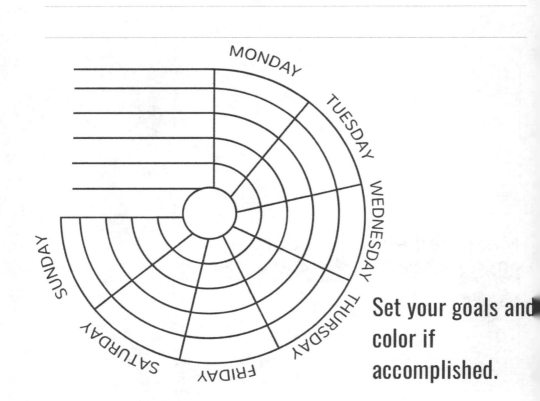

Set your goals and color if accomplished.

FITNESS TRACKER
Meals

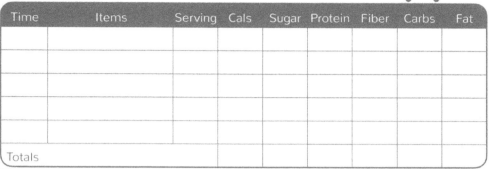

Time	Items	Serving	Cals	Sugar	Protein	Fiber	Carbs	Fat
Totals								

Exercise

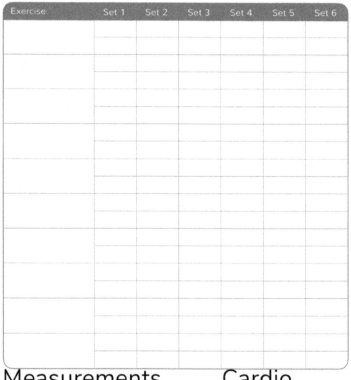

Exercise	Set 1	Set 2	Set 3	Set 4	Set 5	Set 6

Water Tracker

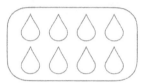

Notes:

Measurements

Measurements	
Neck	
Chest	
Bicep	
Waist	
Hips	
Thigh	
Calf	

Cardio

Exercise	Time	Intensity	Cals

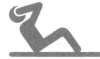

FITNESS TRACKER

Meals

Time	Items	Serving	Cals	Sugar	Protein	Fiber	Carbs	Fat
Totals								

Exercise

Exercise	Set 1	Set 2	Set 3	Set 4	Set 5	Set 6

Water Tracker

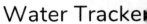
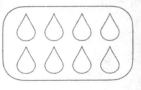

Notes:

Measurements

Measurements	
Neck	
Chest	
Bicep	
Waist	
Hips	
Thigh	
Calf	

Cardio

Exercise	Time	Intensity	Cals

FITNESS TRACKER
Meals

Time	Items	Serving	Cals	Sugar	Protein	Fiber	Carbs	Fat
Totals								

Exercise

Water Tracker

Notes:

Exercise	Set 1	Set 2	Set 3	Set 4	Set 5	Set 6

Measurements

Cardio

Measurements	
Neck	
Chest	
Bicep	
Waist	
Hips	
Thigh	
Calf	

Exercise	Time	Intensity	Cals

FITNESS TRACKER
Meals

Time	Items	Serving	Cals	Sugar	Protein	Fiber	Carbs	Fat
Totals								

Exercise

Water Tracker

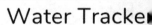

Exercise	Set 1	Set 2	Set 3	Set 4	Set 5	Set 6

Notes:

Measurements   Cardio

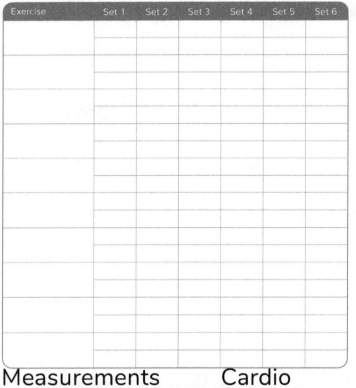

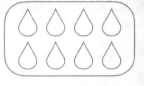

FITNESS TRACKER

Meals

Time	Items	Serving	Cals	Sugar	Protein	Fiber	Carbs	Fat
Totals								

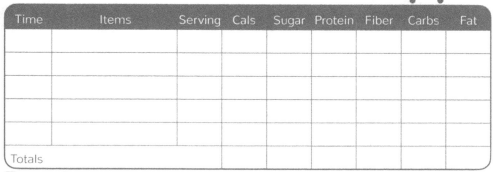

Exercise

Exercise	Set 1	Set 2	Set 3	Set 4	Set 5	Set 6

Water Tracker

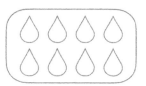

Notes:

Measurements

Measurements	
Neck	
Chest	
Bicep	
Waist	
Hips	
Thigh	
Calf	

Cardio

Exercise	Time	Intensity	Cals

FITNESS TRACKER

Meals

Time	Items	Serving	Cals	Sugar	Protein	Fiber	Carbs	Fat
Totals								

Exercise

Exercise	Set 1	Set 2	Set 3	Set 4	Set 5	Set 6

Water Tracker

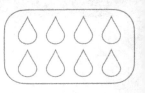

Notes:

Measurements

Measurements	
Neck	
Chest	
Bicep	
Waist	
Hips	
Thigh	
Calf	

Cardio

Exercise	Time	Intensity	Cals

FITNESS TRACKER

Meals

Time	Items	Serving	Cals	Sugar	Protein	Fiber	Carbs	Fat
Totals								

Exercise

Exercise	Set 1	Set 2	Set 3	Set 4	Set 5	Set 6

Water Tracker

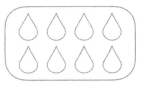

Notes:

Measurements

Measurements	
Neck	
Chest	
Bicep	
Waist	
Hips	
Thigh	
Calf	

Cardio

Exercise	Time	Intensity	Cals

WEEKLY NOTES

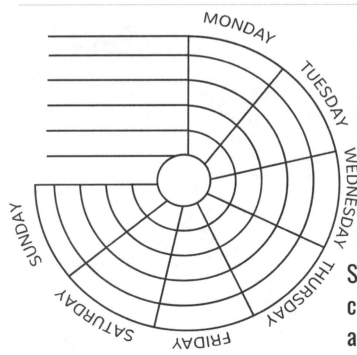

Set your goals and color if accomplished.

FITNESS TRACKER
Meals

Time	Items	Serving	Cals	Sugar	Protein	Fiber	Carbs	Fat
Totals								

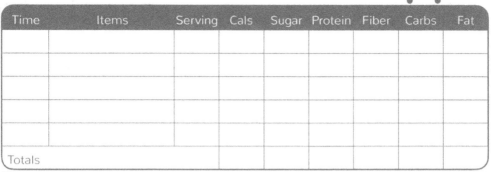

Exercise

Exercise	Set 1	Set 2	Set 3	Set 4	Set 5	Set 6

Water Tracker

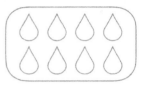

Notes:

Measurements

Measurements	
Neck	
Chest	
Bicep	
Waist	
Hips	
Thigh	
Calf	

Cardio

Exercise	Time	Intensity	Cals

FITNESS TRACKER

Meals

Time	Items	Serving	Cals	Sugar	Protein	Fiber	Carbs	Fat
Totals								

Exercise

Exercise	Set 1	Set 2	Set 3	Set 4	Set 5	Set 6

Water Tracker

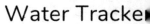

Notes:

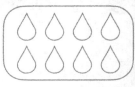

Measurements

Measurements	
Neck	
Chest	
Bicep	
Waist	
Hips	
Thigh	
Calf	

Cardio

Exercise	Time	Intensity	Cals

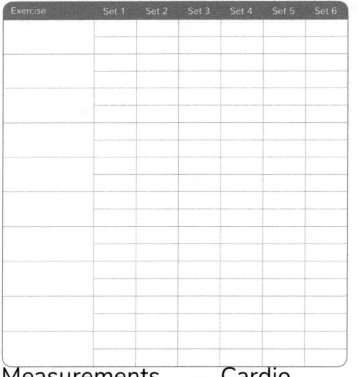

FITNESS TRACKER

Meals

Time	Items	Serving	Cals	Sugar	Protein	Fiber	Carbs	Fat
Totals								

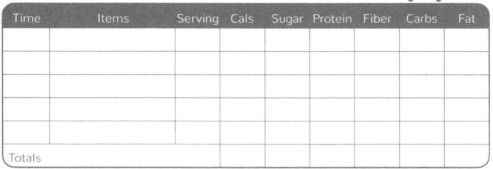

Exercise

Exercise	Set 1	Set 2	Set 3	Set 4	Set 5	Set 6

Water Tracker

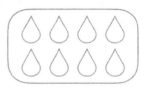

Notes:

Measurements

Measurements	
Neck	
Chest	
Bicep	
Waist	
Hips	
Thigh	
Calf	

Cardio

Exercise	Time	Intensity	Cals

FITNESS TRACKER

Meals

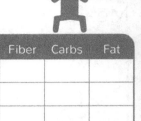

Time	Items	Serving	Cals	Sugar	Protein	Fiber	Carbs	Fat
Totals								

Exercise

Water Tracker

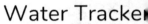

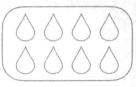

Exercise	Set 1	Set 2	Set 3	Set 4	Set 5	Set 6

Notes:

Measurements

Cardio

Measurements	
Neck	
Chest	
Bicep	
Waist	
Hips	
Thigh	
Calf	

Exercise	Time	Intensity	Cals

FITNESS TRACKER
Meals

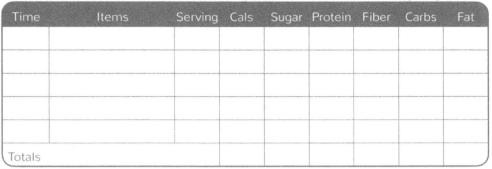

Time	Items	Serving	Cals	Sugar	Protein	Fiber	Carbs	Fat
Totals								

Exercise

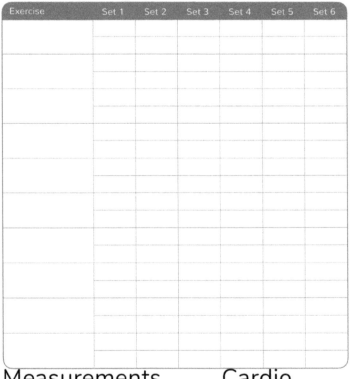

Exercise	Set 1	Set 2	Set 3	Set 4	Set 5	Set 6

Water Tracker

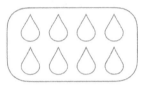

Notes:

Measurements

Measurements	
Neck	
Chest	
Bicep	
Waist	
Hips	
Thigh	
Calf	

Cardio

Exercise	Time	Intensity	Cals

FITNESS TRACKER
Meals

Time	Items	Serving	Cals	Sugar	Protein	Fiber	Carbs	Fat
Totals								

Exercise

Exercise	Set 1	Set 2	Set 3	Set 4	Set 5	Set 6

Water Tracker

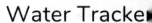

Notes:

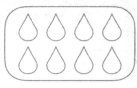

Measurements

Measurements	
Neck	
Chest	
Bicep	
Waist	
Hips	
Thigh	
Calf	

Cardio

Exercise	Time	Intensity	Cals

FITNESS TRACKER
Meals

Time	Items	Serving	Cals	Sugar	Protein	Fiber	Carbs	Fat
Totals								

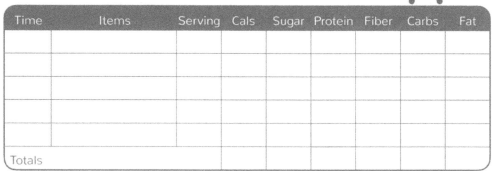

Exercise

Exercise	Set 1	Set 2	Set 3	Set 4	Set 5	Set 6

Water Tracker

Notes:

Measurements

Measurements	
Neck	
Chest	
Bicep	
Waist	
Hips	
Thigh	
Calf	

Cardio

Exercise	Time	Intensity	Cals

WEEKLY NOTES

Set your goals and color if accomplished.

FITNESS TRACKER

Meals

Time	Items	Serving	Cals	Sugar	Protein	Fiber	Carbs	Fat
Totals								

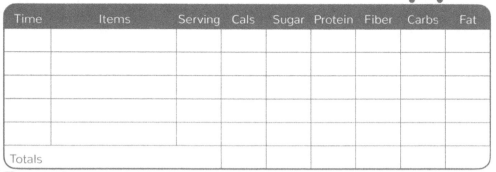

Exercise

Exercise	Set 1	Set 2	Set 3	Set 4	Set 5	Set 6

Water Tracker

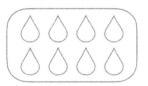

Notes:

Measurements

Measurements	
Neck	
Chest	
Bicep	
Waist	
Hips	
Thigh	
Calf	

Cardio

Exercise	Time	Intensity	Cals

FITNESS TRACKER

Meals

Time	Items	Serving	Cals	Sugar	Protein	Fiber	Carbs	Fat
Totals								

Exercise

Water Tracker

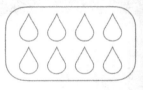

Exercise	Set 1	Set 2	Set 3	Set 4	Set 5	Set 6

Notes:

Measurements

Cardio

Measurements	
Neck	
Chest	
Bicep	
Waist	
Hips	
Thigh	
Calf	

Exercise	Time	Intensity	Cals

FITNESS TRACKER
Meals

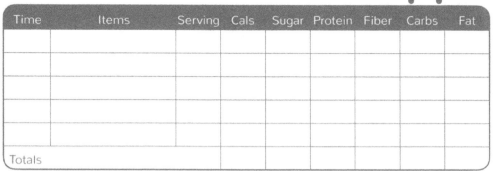

Time	Items	Serving	Cals	Sugar	Protein	Fiber	Carbs	Fat
Totals								

Exercise

Water Tracker

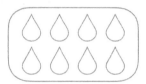

Exercise	Set 1	Set 2	Set 3	Set 4	Set 5	Set 6

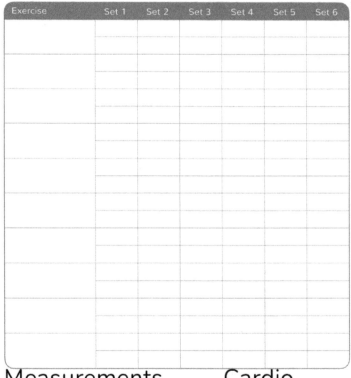

Notes:

Measurements

Measurements	
Neck	
Chest	
Bicep	
Waist	
Hips	
Thigh	
Calf	

Cardio

Exercise	Time	Intensity	Cals

FITNESS TRACKER

Meals

Time	Items	Serving	Cals	Sugar	Protein	Fiber	Carbs	Fat
Totals								

Exercise

Exercise	Set 1	Set 2	Set 3	Set 4	Set 5	Set 6

Water Tracker

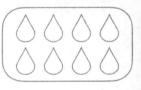

Notes:

_____
_____
_____
_____
_____
_____
_____
_____
_____
_____
_____
_____
_____
_____

Measurements

Measurements	
Neck	
Chest	
Bicep	
Waist	
Hips	
Thigh	
Calf	

Cardio

Exercise	Time	Intensity	Cals

FITNESS TRACKER

Meals

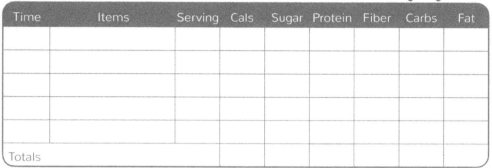

Time	Items	Serving	Cals	Sugar	Protein	Fiber	Carbs	Fat
Totals								

Exercise

Exercise	Set 1	Set 2	Set 3	Set 4	Set 5	Set 6

Water Tracker

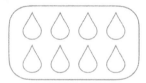

Notes:

Measurements

Measurements	
Neck	
Chest	
Bicep	
Waist	
Hips	
Thigh	
Calf	

Cardio

Exercise	Time	Intensity	Cals

FITNESS TRACKER
Meals

Time	Items	Serving	Cals	Sugar	Protein	Fiber	Carbs	Fat
Totals								

Exercise

Water Tracker

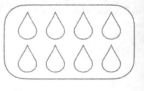

Exercise	Set 1	Set 2	Set 3	Set 4	Set 5	Set 6

Notes:

Measurements

Measurements	
Neck	
Chest	
Bicep	
Waist	
Hips	
Thigh	
Calf	

Cardio

Exercise	Time	Intensity	Cals

FITNESS TRACKER
Meals

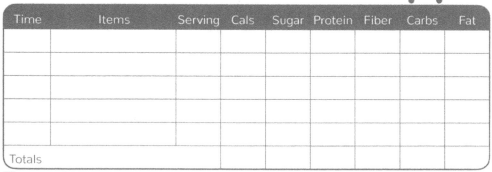

Time	Items	Serving	Cals	Sugar	Protein	Fiber	Carbs	Fat
Totals								

Exercise

Water Tracker

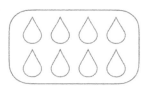

Exercise	Set 1	Set 2	Set 3	Set 4	Set 5	Set 6

Notes:

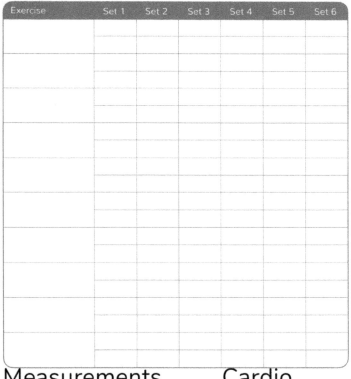

Measurements

Cardio

Measurements	
Neck	
Chest	
Bicep	
Waist	
Hips	
Thigh	
Calf	

Exercise	Time	Intensity	Cals

WEEKLY NOTES

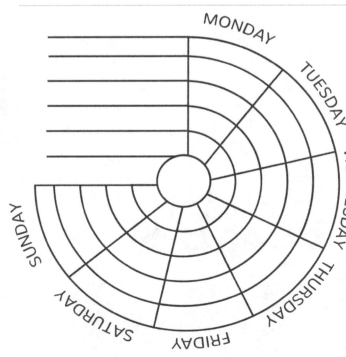

Set your goals and color if accomplished.

FITNESS TRACKER
Meals

Time	Items	Serving	Cals	Sugar	Protein	Fiber	Carbs	Fat
Totals								

Exercise

Exercise	Set 1	Set 2	Set 3	Set 4	Set 5	Set 6

Water Tracker

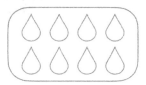

Notes:

Measurements

Measurements	
Neck	
Chest	
Bicep	
Waist	
Hips	
Thigh	
Calf	

Cardio

Exercise	Time	Intensity	Cals

FITNESS TRACKER
Meals

Time	Items	Serving	Cals	Sugar	Protein	Fiber	Carbs	Fat
Totals								

Exercise

Water Tracker

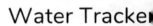

Exercise	Set 1	Set 2	Set 3	Set 4	Set 5	Set 6

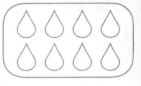

Notes:

Measurements

Cardio

Measurements	
Neck	
Chest	
Bicep	
Waist	
Hips	
Thigh	
Calf	

Exercise	Time	Intensity	Cals

FITNESS TRACKER
Meals

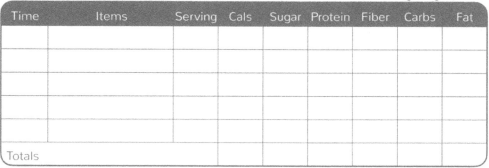

Time	Items	Serving	Cals	Sugar	Protein	Fiber	Carbs	Fat
Totals								

Exercise

Water Tracker

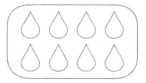

Exercise	Set 1	Set 2	Set 3	Set 4	Set 5	Set 6

Notes:

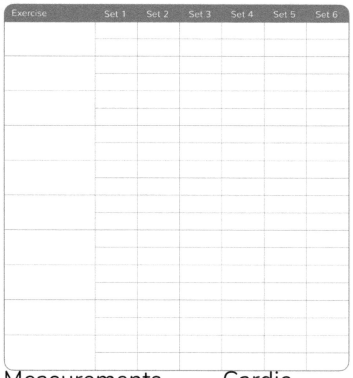

Measurements

Cardio

Measurements	
Neck	
Chest	
Bicep	
Waist	
Hips	
Thigh	
Calf	

Exercise	Time	Intensity	Cals

FITNESS TRACKER
Meals

Time	Items	Serving	Cals	Sugar	Protein	Fiber	Carbs	Fat
Totals								

Exercise

Water Tracker

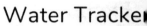

Exercise	Set 1	Set 2	Set 3	Set 4	Set 5	Set 6

Notes:

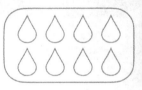

Measurements

Cardio

Measurements	
Neck	
Chest	
Bicep	
Waist	
Hips	
Thigh	
Calf	

Exercise	Time	Intensity	Cals

FITNESS TRACKER

Meals

Time	Items	Serving	Cals	Sugar	Protein	Fiber	Carbs	Fat
Totals								

Exercise

Exercise	Set 1	Set 2	Set 3	Set 4	Set 5	Set 6

Water Tracker

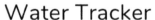

Notes:

Measurements

Measurements	
Neck	
Chest	
Bicep	
Waist	
Hips	
Thigh	
Calf	

Cardio

Exercise	Time	Intensity	Cals

FITNESS TRACKER
Meals

Time	Items	Serving	Cals	Sugar	Protein	Fiber	Carbs	Fat
Totals								

Exercise

Exercise	Set 1	Set 2	Set 3	Set 4	Set 5	Set 6

Water Tracker

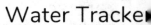

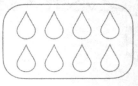

Notes:

Measurements

Measurements	
Neck	
Chest	
Bicep	
Waist	
Hips	
Thigh	
Calf	

Cardio

Exercise	Time	Intensity	Cals

FITNESS TRACKER
Meals

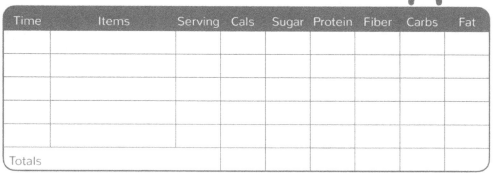

Time	Items	Serving	Cals	Sugar	Protein	Fiber	Carbs	Fat
Totals								

Exercise

Water Tracker

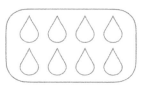

Exercise	Set 1	Set 2	Set 3	Set 4	Set 5	Set 6

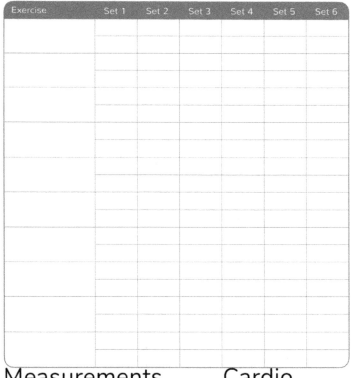

Notes:

Measurements

Cardio

Measurements	
Neck	
Chest	
Bicep	
Waist	
Hips	
Thigh	
Calf	

Exercise	Time	Intensity	Cals

WEEKLY NOTES

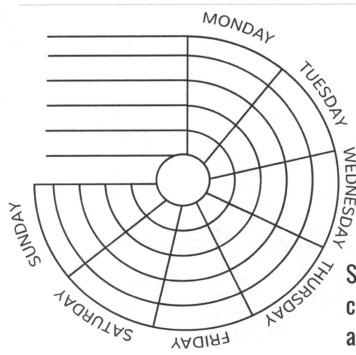

Set your goals and color if accomplished.

FITNESS TRACKER

Meals

Time	Items	Serving	Cals	Sugar	Protein	Fiber	Carbs	Fat
Totals								

Exercise

Exercise	Set 1	Set 2	Set 3	Set 4	Set 5	Set 6

Water Tracker

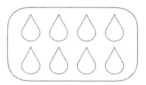

Notes:

Measurements

Measurements	
Neck	
Chest	
Bicep	
Waist	
Hips	
Thigh	
Calf	

Cardio

Exercise	Time	Intensity	Cals

FITNESS TRACKER
Meals

Time	Items	Serving	Cals	Sugar	Protein	Fiber	Carbs	Fat
Totals								

Exercise

Exercise	Set 1	Set 2	Set 3	Set 4	Set 5	Set 6

Water Tracker

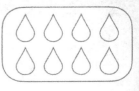

Notes:

Measurements

Measurements	
Neck	
Chest	
Bicep	
Waist	
Hips	
Thigh	
Calf	

Cardio

Exercise	Time	Intensity	Cals

FITNESS TRACKER
Meals

Time	Items	Serving	Cals	Sugar	Protein	Fiber	Carbs	Fat
Totals								

Exercise

Exercise	Set 1	Set 2	Set 3	Set 4	Set 5	Set 6

Water Tracker

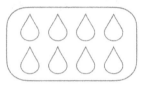

Notes:

Measurements

Measurements	
Neck	
Chest	
Bicep	
Waist	
Hips	
Thigh	
Calf	

Cardio

Exercise	Time	Intensity	Cals

FITNESS TRACKER

Meals

Time	Items	Serving	Cals	Sugar	Protein	Fiber	Carbs	Fat
Totals								

Exercise

Exercise	Set 1	Set 2	Set 3	Set 4	Set 5	Set 6

Water Tracker

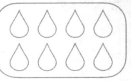

Notes:

Measurements

Measurements	
Neck	
Chest	
Bicep	
Waist	
Hips	
Thigh	
Calf	

Cardio

Exercise	Time	Intensity	Cals

FITNESS TRACKER

Meals

Time	Items	Serving	Cals	Sugar	Protein	Fiber	Carbs	Fat
Totals								

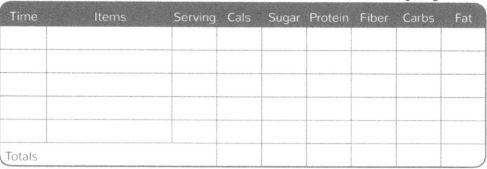

Exercise

Exercise	Set 1	Set 2	Set 3	Set 4	Set 5	Set 6

Water Tracker

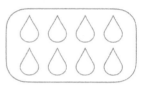

Notes:

Measurements

Measurements	
Neck	
Chest	
Bicep	
Waist	
Hips	
Thigh	
Calf	

Cardio

Exercise	Time	Intensity	Cals

FITNESS TRACKER

Meals

Time	Items	Serving	Cals	Sugar	Protein	Fiber	Carbs	Fat
Totals								

Exercise

Exercise	Set 1	Set 2	Set 3	Set 4	Set 5	Set 6

Water Tracker

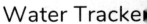

Notes:

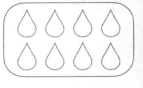

Measurements

Measurements	
Neck	
Chest	
Bicep	
Waist	
Hips	
Thigh	
Calf	

Cardio

Exercise	Time	Intensity	Cals

FITNESS TRACKER

Meals

Time	Items	Serving	Cals	Sugar	Protein	Fiber	Carbs	Fat
Totals								

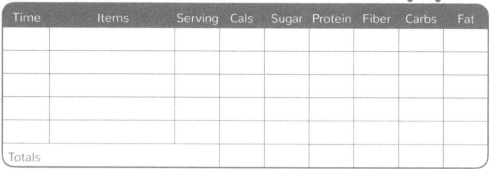

Exercise

Exercise	Set 1	Set 2	Set 3	Set 4	Set 5	Set 6

Water Tracker

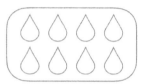

Notes:

Measurements

Measurements	
Neck	
Chest	
Bicep	
Waist	
Hips	
Thigh	
Calf	

Cardio

Exercise	Time	Intensity	Cals

WEEKLY NOTES

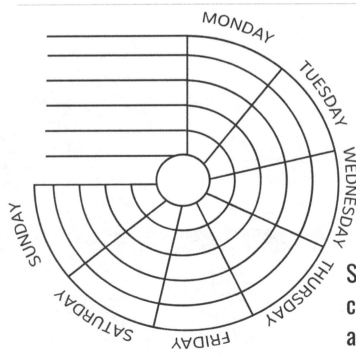

Set your goals and color if accomplished.

FITNESS TRACKER
Meals

Time	Items	Serving	Cals	Sugar	Protein	Fiber	Carbs	Fat
Totals								

Exercise

Exercise	Set 1	Set 2	Set 3	Set 4	Set 5	Set 6

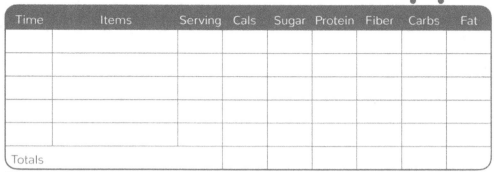

Water Tracker

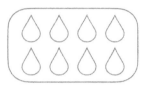

Notes:

Measurements

Measurements	
Neck	
Chest	
Bicep	
Waist	
Hips	
Thigh	
Calf	

Cardio

Exercise	Time	Intensity	Cals

FITNESS TRACKER

Meals

Time	Items	Serving	Cals	Sugar	Protein	Fiber	Carbs	Fat
Totals								

Exercise

Exercise	Set 1	Set 2	Set 3	Set 4	Set 5	Set 6

Water Tracker

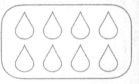

Notes:

Measurements

Measurements	
Neck	
Chest	
Bicep	
Waist	
Hips	
Thigh	
Calf	

Cardio

Exercise	Time	Intensity	Cals

FITNESS TRACKER
Meals

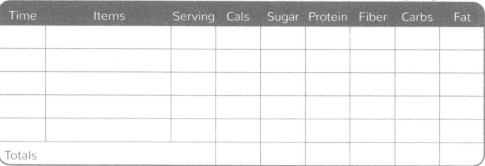

Time	Items	Serving	Cals	Sugar	Protein	Fiber	Carbs	Fat
Totals								

Exercise

Water Tracker

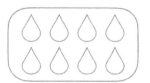

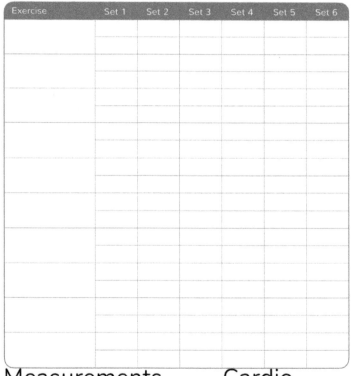

Exercise	Set 1	Set 2	Set 3	Set 4	Set 5	Set 6

Notes:

Measurements

Measurements	
Neck	
Chest	
Bicep	
Waist	
Hips	
Thigh	
Calf	

Cardio

Exercise	Time	Intensity	Cals

FITNESS TRACKER

Meals

Time	Items	Serving	Cals	Sugar	Protein	Fiber	Carbs	Fat
Totals								

Exercise

Exercise	Set 1	Set 2	Set 3	Set 4	Set 5	Set 6

Water Tracker

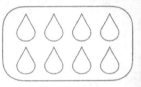

Notes:

_____
_____
_____
_____
_____
_____
_____
_____
_____
_____
_____
_____
_____
_____
_____
_____

Measurements

Measurements	
Neck	
Chest	
Bicep	
Waist	
Hips	
Thigh	
Calf	

Cardio

Exercise	Time	Intensity	Cals

FITNESS TRACKER

Meals

Time	Items	Serving	Cals	Sugar	Protein	Fiber	Carbs	Fat
Totals								

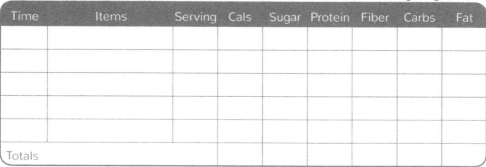

Exercise

Exercise	Set 1	Set 2	Set 3	Set 4	Set 5	Set 6

Water Tracker

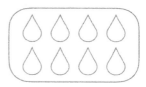

Notes:

Measurements

Measurements	
Neck	
Chest	
Bicep	
Waist	
Hips	
Thigh	
Calf	

Cardio

Exercise	Time	Intensity	Cals

FITNESS TRACKER

Meals

Time	Items	Serving	Cals	Sugar	Protein	Fiber	Carbs	Fat
Totals								

Exercise

Exercise	Set 1	Set 2	Set 3	Set 4	Set 5	Set 6

Water Tracker

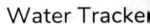
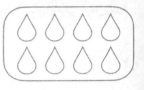

Notes:

Measurements

Measurements	
Neck	
Chest	
Bicep	
Waist	
Hips	
Thigh	
Calf	

Cardio

Exercise	Time	Intensity	Cals

FITNESS TRACKER
Meals

Time	Items	Serving	Cals	Sugar	Protein	Fiber	Carbs	Fat
Totals								

Exercise

Water Tracker

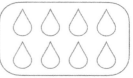

Exercise	Set 1	Set 2	Set 3	Set 4	Set 5	Set 6

Notes:

Measurements   Cardio

Measurements	
Neck	
Chest	
Bicep	
Waist	
Hips	
Thigh	
Calf	

Exercise	Time	Intensity	Cals

WEEKLY NOTES

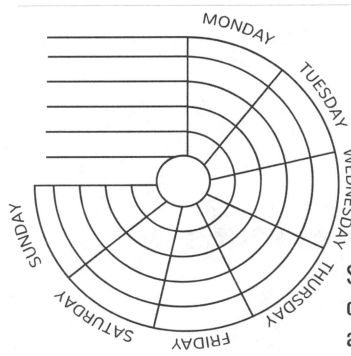

Set your goals and color if accomplished.

FITNESS TRACKER

Meals

Time	Items	Serving	Cals	Sugar	Protein	Fiber	Carbs	Fat
Totals								

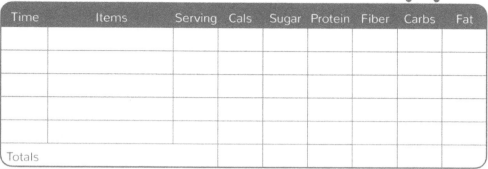

Exercise

Exercise	Set 1	Set 2	Set 3	Set 4	Set 5	Set 6

Water Tracker

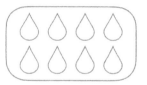

Notes:

Measurements

Measurements	
Neck	
Chest	
Bicep	
Waist	
Hips	
Thigh	
Calf	

Cardio

Exercise	Time	Intensity	Cals

FITNESS TRACKER
Meals

Time	Items	Serving	Cals	Sugar	Protein	Fiber	Carbs	Fat
Totals								

Exercise

Water Tracker

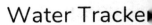

Exercise	Set 1	Set 2	Set 3	Set 4	Set 5	Set 6

Notes:

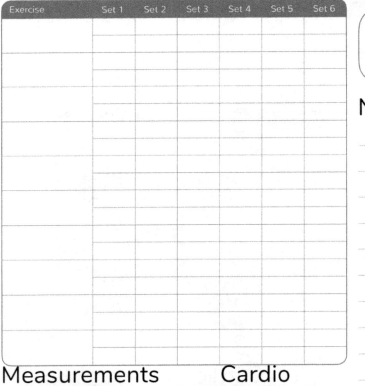

Measurements

Cardio

Measurements	
Neck	
Chest	
Bicep	
Waist	
Hips	
Thigh	
Calf	

Exercise	Time	Intensity	Cals

FITNESS TRACKER
Meals

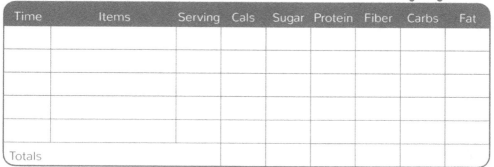

Time	Items	Serving	Cals	Sugar	Protein	Fiber	Carbs	Fat
Totals								

Exercise

Water Tracker

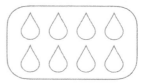

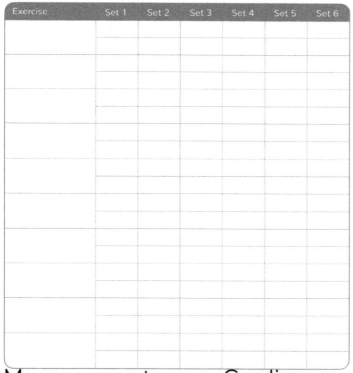

Exercise	Set 1	Set 2	Set 3	Set 4	Set 5	Set 6

Notes:

Measurements

Cardio

Measurements	
Neck	
Chest	
Bicep	
Waist	
Hips	
Thigh	
Calf	

Exercise	Time	Intensity	Cals

FITNESS TRACKER

Meals

Time	Items	Serving	Cals	Sugar	Protein	Fiber	Carbs	Fat
Totals								

Exercise

Exercise	Set 1	Set 2	Set 3	Set 4	Set 5	Set 6

Water Tracker

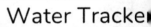

Notes:

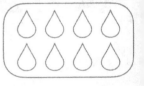

Measurements

Measurements	
Neck	
Chest	
Bicep	
Waist	
Hips	
Thigh	
Calf	

Cardio

Exercise	Time	Intensity	Cals

FITNESS TRACKER
Meals

Time	Items	Serving	Cals	Sugar	Protein	Fiber	Carbs	Fat
Totals								

Exercise

Exercise	Set 1	Set 2	Set 3	Set 4	Set 5	Set 6

Water Tracker

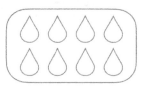

Notes:

Measurements

Measurements	
Neck	
Chest	
Bicep	
Waist	
Hips	
Thigh	
Calf	

Cardio

Exercise	Time	Intensity	Cals

FITNESS TRACKER

Meals

Time	Items	Serving	Cals	Sugar	Protein	Fiber	Carbs	Fat
Totals								

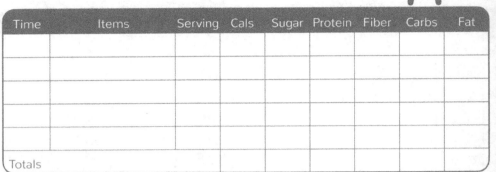

Exercise

Exercise	Set 1	Set 2	Set 3	Set 4	Set 5	Set 6

Water Tracker

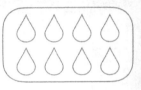

Notes:

Measurements

Measurements	
Neck	
Chest	
Bicep	
Waist	
Hips	
Thigh	
Calf	

Cardio

Exercise	Time	Intensity	Cals

FITNESS TRACKER

Meals

Time	Items	Serving	Cals	Sugar	Protein	Fiber	Carbs	Fat
Totals								

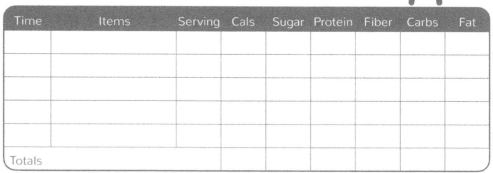

Exercise

Exercise	Set 1	Set 2	Set 3	Set 4	Set 5	Set 6

Water Tracker

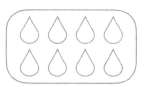

Notes:

Measurements

Measurements	
Neck	
Chest	
Bicep	
Waist	
Hips	
Thigh	
Calf	

Cardio

Exercise	Time	Intensity	Cals

WEEKLY NOTES

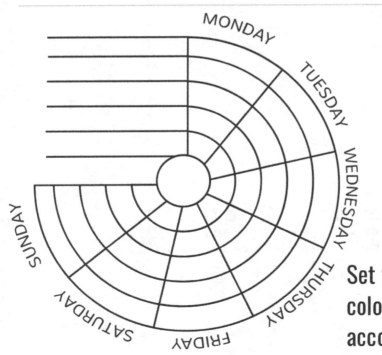

Set your goals and color if accomplished.

We hope
you enjoyed our book !

Our goal, as a small family company is making your experience a great one.
There's nothing better than reading the valuable feedback from you,
so please let us know if you like our book at :
eightidd@gmail.com
or leave a review with your thoughts about it.

Thanks for your amazing support !

CPSIA information can be obtained
at www.ICGtesting.com
Printed in the USA
LVHW021553230121
677175LV00003B/205